Infant Massage Guide Guide Made Simple:

Full Guide on How to Massage Your Baby Proficiently;Its Types, Benefits & Set Up; How to Massage & Mistakes to Avoid & Quiz for You & Lots More

By

Dr. Bradley L. Jackson

Copyright@2020

TABLE OF CONTENTS

CHAPTER ONE

INTRODUCTION

Baby Massage

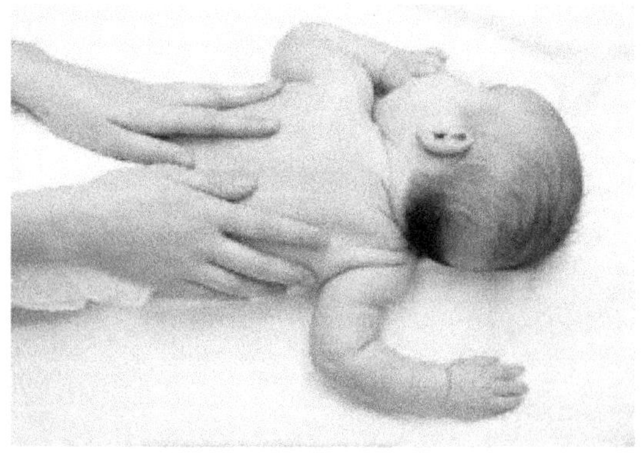

Baby massage as it is the modus operandi of rubbing baby muscles as well as stroking the baby's body in a mode expressly designed for them.

Administering your baby timely

massages is perfect for his/her poignant well-being as well. Caring touch and rhythmic movement are among the most powerful forms of communication between infants and their parents, so they are great ways for you to bond.

Besides, you need at last 10-15 minutes. You can start a massage when you're relaxed and your baby is silent but alert.(If you try to massage a fussy infant, you may overstimulate and make him even unhappy). Start after changing a diaper or as part of bedtime routine.

CHAPTER TWO

Types of Baby Massage

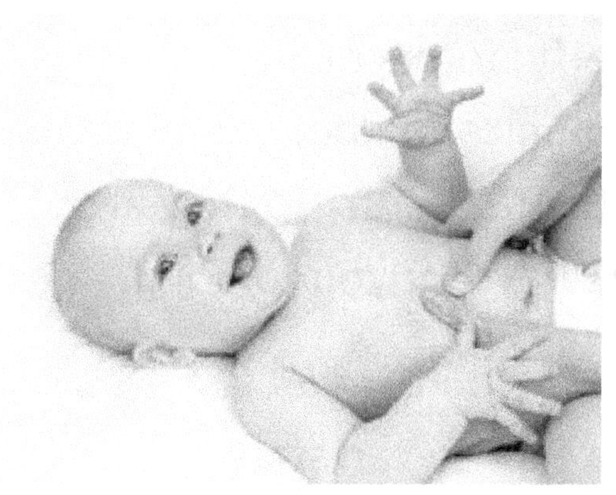

Belly massage

Your hands should be placed at the level of your baby's navel. Rub your fingertips gently and firmly over his tummy in a circular motion. Repeat the process.

Leg Massage

Softly but firmly wrap your hands around your baby's leg and slide your hands down from thigh to the ankle. It should be done few times; do same to the other leg.

Neck Massage

With one hand support your baby's head. The thumb of your other hand should be placed on one side of her neck and your first two fingers on the other side. With your fingertips softly rub your baby's neck in a circular motion.

Arm Massage

Between your hands softly roll your baby's arm, starting from the shoulder down to the wrist. Repeat the process two to three times, and then switch to the other arm.

Hold me Close

The skin-to-skin contact is good for all infants, but it's particularly helpful for babies born prematurely. That is why *"kangaroo care"* is encourage by most neonatal intensive care units where the mother place her preemie on her bare chest, holding her tummy-to-tummy. "This type of body contact with the baby relaxes a preterm infant and can help her grow,'' it was said by Susan Ludington, Ph.D., a professor of pediatric nursing at case western reserve University, in Cleveland, who has studied kangaroo care lengthily.

Colic- - Relief Massage

You give your baby a belly massage. After that you bend his knees up to his tummy and you hold it for about 30 seconds before releasing. This process should be repeated. The edge of one of your hand should be placed on your baby's tummy, gliding from the tummy button down in a rhythmic pattern, this

process help to release pent – up
gas.

CHAPTER THREE

What are the benefits of Baby Massage?

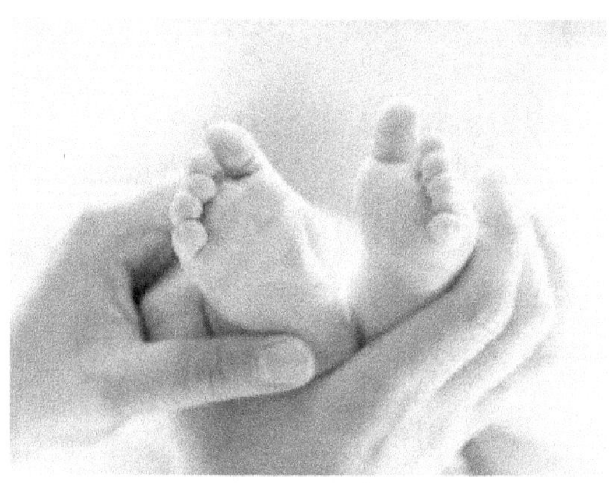

There are several natural benefits of baby massage, they are:

Stimulate Nervous System:

Massage is very important to the baby's nervous system since your baby's motor skills development is improved by massage.

It Helps Baby to Sleep Well:

Infants sleep better when they are massaged. Infants who are massaged before going to bed **produces a sleep regulator hormone called melatonin.** Massage has several benefits of faster muscles gain to increase immune response.

Relaxes the Muscles, Relieves Stress:

Massage helps relax infant muscles, and stimulate growth. It relieves stress in babies by stimulating the release of oxytocin, a feeling goodneurohormone, and reduces a stress hormone called cortisol.

It Helps to Improve Blood Circulation:

Massage improves the circulation of blood and also reduces the level of discomfort caused by teething, gas or acidity, and congestion. It benefits the digestive system by stimulates the nerves that pass through the digestive tract.

My Increase the Quality of Life for Differently-Abled Infants:

Massage helps to soothe infants with cerebral palsy or Down's syndrome. When premature infants are massage regularly they show better motor development. They show to gain more weight faster than premature infants that are never massaged.

Massage Boosts Psychological and Social Development:

Stimulation of the infant sense of touch has an advantage on the baby's psychological and social development along with strengthening the bond with the parent and their baby's.

CHAPTER FOUR

Setup for Massage

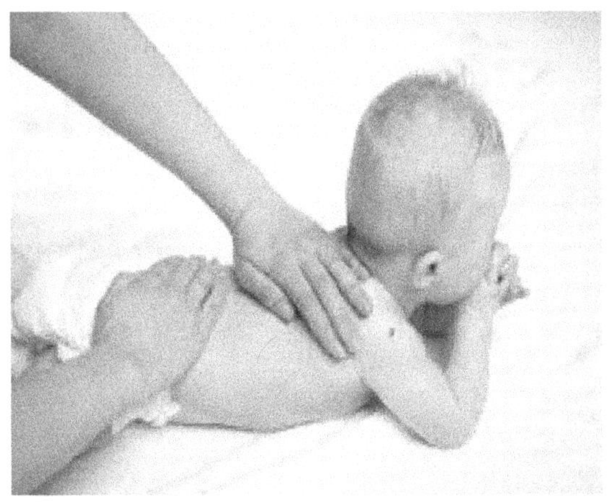

Before you begin the process of massaging your baby, you need to set up various things.

Sit on a soft carpeted floor or on a bed. Place a towel in front of you. A towel can also be placed on a table to massage your baby while you stand. The excess oil are absorb by the towel.

A Comfortable Room Temperature Should be Maintained. During summers you must ensure there is sufficientcirculation of cool and fresh air in the room and during winters, you must make sure that the room is warm.

Good Lighting System. It is very important to have lighting in the room and use as much as possible.

Select Massaging oil that is made exactly for Babies.

Choose unscented oils, with natural scents and no perfumes, so that no problem will arise even if the oil is ingested by mistake. You can consult your pediatrician to know about the most suitable oil for your baby.

You can decide to Massage Your Baby With or Without the Nappy.

When massaging your baby's tummy you can loosen it. Massaging without nappy may upsurge the risk of accidental soiling, but it makes sure every part of the baby's body is massage.

CHAPTER FIVE

How to Massage Your Baby

Here are step-by-step guide on how to massage your baby in the right way:

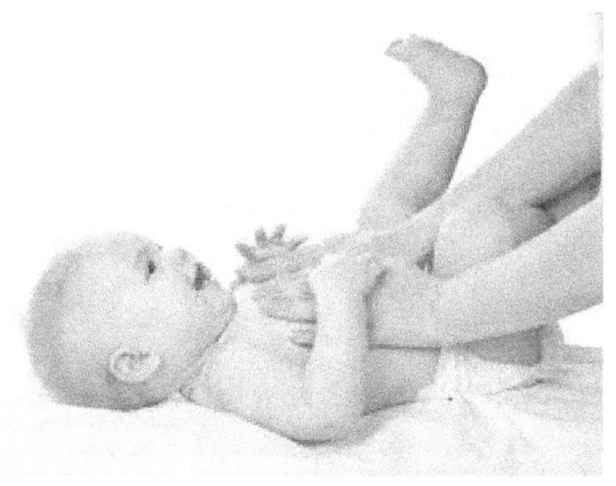

Step 1: Seek the Baby's permission

Firstly, you have to seek your baby's permission since you would not like to massage when they are not interested. The easy way to do this is to take little oil in your palms and you gently rub it on your baby's tummy and behind the ears and you observe your baby's body language. If the baby shows positive signs with what you are doing, then you can continue with the massage. If the baby being touched and cries when massaging, then it is not the right time yet to massage your baby.

Have it in mind that, initially, since the experience is new your baby may seem uncomfortable with the massage. Resistance becomes less as they get used to it, and your baby may start to enjoy it.

Step 2: Massage the Legs

Start with your baby's feet. Rub little oil in your palm and massage the soles. Use your thumb to massage the heel up to the toe. Slowly, make circles with your thumb all over the bottom of each foot and the toes. Avoid pulling of toe like they do in adult massage. Instead, massage the toe lightly rightly to the tip.

You can massage both legs at once if your baby is calm and relaxed or you can lift one at a time. You lift one of the legs and make a softly strokes on the ankle and slowly extend it close to the thighs.

End your leg massage by gently grasping the thighs with both hands. Then you gently stroke toward the heart from foot to thigh.

Step 3: Move to the Arms

The pattern of massaging the arm is quite similar to that of the legs. You hold your baby's hands and make circular strokes on both palms. Gently make small strokes on the baby's fingers, and move towards the finger tips.

You turn the baby's hand around and softly massage the back of the hand with straight strokes near the wrist. Then, softly massage the wrists in a circular motion.

Lastly move your strokes slowly towards the forearm and then towards the upper arm. You massage the entire arm with softly circular motions as if you are wringing a towel.

Step 4: Massage the Chest and Shoulder

A gentle stroke should be made in tandem from the right and left shoulder near the chest of the baby. Then you trace your hand back to the shoulder. Slowly repeat the motion. Then, place both your hands at the middle of your baby's chest and rub outwards from the body near the lateral side.

Create softly strokes outwards from the bottom of the sternum, as if you are tracing the shape of the heart.

Step 5: Massage the Tummy

Remember, the baby's tummy is a delicate area, and so you must avoid even the slightest of pressures. You begin your stroke from the top belly right under the chest bone. Place your palm softly under the chest bone and make clockwise circular strokes across the tummy – all round the belly button. Gently let your hands glide across the belly and do not apply any force.

Avoid the belly button and continue the circular motions in a clockwise direction. In little babies, the belly button/navel can be sensitive and delicate since they have lately shed their umbilical cord stub.

Step 6: Face and Head Massage

Baby's moves a lot this makes massage of the head to be challenging. Start by placing the tip of your index finger at the middle of your baby's forehead and gently stroking along the outline of the face near the chin. From the chin, move your finger near the cheeks and massage the cheeks slowly in a circular motion.

After the face massage, begin with the scalp massage with the fingertip like you are shampooing your baby's hair.

Ensure you are using gentle pressure from your finger tip and make sure you do not apply any extra force since the baby's skull is delicate.

Massage your baby's forehead softly by moving your fingers outwards from the middle of the forehead.

Step 7: Back Massage

Turn your baby around and massage the back. Your baby's hand should be placed outstretched on the tummy with the hands at the front and not on the sides.

Put your fingertips on the baby's upper back and trace clockwise circles while you are moving the strokes gently towards the buttocks.

You then put your middle and index finger on either side of the upper spine and slowly move the finger down to the buttocks. Make sure your fingers are not on the spine. Instead, put two fingers on either side of the spinal groove and run them down.

CHAPTER SIX

Common Massage Mistakes You Must Avoid

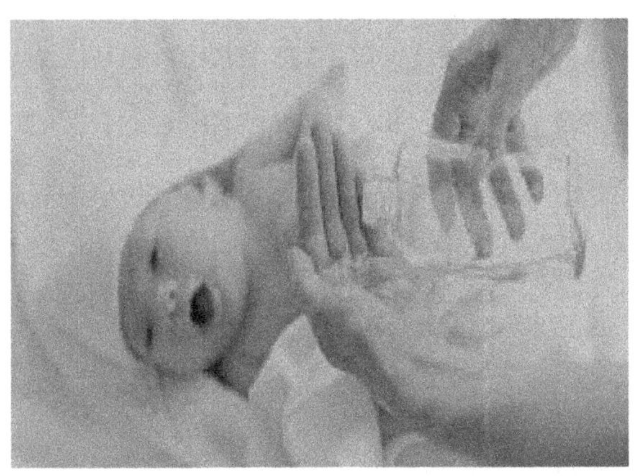

Massaging Your Baby Forcefully

Always remember your baby is delicate and cannot handle a lot of pressure on his tender

skinand newly formed bones.
Ensure that the massage is
gentle and comforting.

Massaging Your Baby in the Wrong Position

The position you take when
massaging your baby is very
important. Ensure you are sitting
on a flat, even surface while
massaging your baby. You place
your baby in a soft cloth before
you start the massage. It helps to
prevent your baby from slipping
from your hands and fall on the
ground.

Massaging Your Baby While Doing Something Else

Massaging your little one, while you are engage in other activity is wrong, even if it is something as mundane watching television. Make sure you maintain good eye contact with your kid, talk and smile to your baby lovingly to bond your sweetheart. It will make your baby know how much you enjoy spending time with her.

Massaging against Your Baby's Wishes

Massaging your baby in an irritated state will only stress and frustrate him out. When child displays secret language of any upset refrain from the massage at once. There are several ways to soothe and bond with your baby- and you can schedule another day for your baby massage.

Using Harsh Oils

Harsh as well smelling essential oils such as peppermint and the likes should not be applied on your little one; these oils cause irritation on your very baby's eyes as well as cause your baby bad-tempered and scratchy. It is advisable to use mild and specially formulated oil for your baby's skin.

Wipe Oil from Your Baby's Fingers

Wipe away the oil on your baby's fingers and palms using tissue paper when done with massage. It helps to prevent your baby from accidently ingesting the oil when they place their fingers in their mouth. This is the reason, you choose baby massage oils that are 100% safe for babies and will not result to any health risk even when ingested accidentally.

CHAPTER SEVEN

Quiz for You

Giving your baby regular massages is good for his emotional well-being
TRUE/FALSE

It advisable to massage your baby while engaged in other activities TRUE/FALSE

It is advisable to wipe your baby's finger after a massage TRUE/FALSE

Massage helps to boost psychological and social development of your baby TRUE/FALSE

Massaging your baby forcefully is one of the ways to bond with your baby TRUE/FALSE

Answer

True

False

True

True

False

CHAPTER EIGHT

Take Away

Massage is a great way of improving your bond with your kid while enabling them to develop well. Though, massaging doesn't come naturally to all parents. Do not be discouraged if massaging doesn't work out with your baby at first.

You have to practice few times with your baby before getting it right. The process of practicing helps sdevelop a deeper loving bond with your little one.

The End